DIABETIC DIET COOKBOOK AFTER 50

Healthy & Easy Recipes to Manage and Reverse Diabetic for Seniors

Sheron Johnson

Table of Content

Table of Content 2

INTRODUCTION 4

CHAPTER 1 8

What is Diabetic.. 8

Types of Diabetics 8

Symptoms of Diabetics 9

Preventive Measures for Diabetes 10

CHAPTER 2 14

How to Manage Diabetic Diet 14

Foods to Eat: 14

Foods to Avoid or Limit: 16

Benefit of Diabetic Disease Diet.................................. 17

CHAPTER 3 20

The Power of a Balanced Diet 20

Comprehensive List of Essential Ingredients 22

Risk Factor 25

CHAPTER 4 28

The Plate Method for Balanced Meals..........................28

Portion Sizes for Older Adults.................................28

Meal Plans Samples 29

Chapter 5 34

Recipe 34

Breakfast Recipes..34

Lunch Recipe 43

Dinner Recipe 52

Snack Recipes 61

Dessert and sweet treat.......................................68

Smoothie and Beverages......................................78

CHAPTER 6 86

Success Stories...86

John's Journey to Reversing Diabetes..........................86

Sarah's Success through Dietary Choices 87

Mark's Transformation through Lifestyle Changes 87

Conclusion 90

Meal Planner Journal 92

INTRODUCTION

In a small town nestled between rolling hills, there lived an elderly man named Samuel. He had always been an active and vibrant soul, but as he reached his 70s, he found himself facing a new challenge—diabetes. His doctor had delivered the diagnosis with a heavy heart, urging Samuel to make significant changes to his lifestyle.

One sunny morning, his daughter, Sarah, handed him a copy of the "Diabetic Diet Cookbook After 50." She had heard about it from a friend and thought it might help her father. Samuel, determined to regain control of his health, decided to give it a try.

As he flipped through the pages of the cookbook, he discovered a world of delicious and nutritious recipes tailored to his needs. With each meal he prepared, he learned more about making smart choices in the kitchen. He stocked his pantry with whole grains, lean proteins, and plenty of fresh vegetables.

He started his day with a hearty and filling breakfast of oatmeal with berries and nuts, following one of the cookbook's recipes. He found that his blood sugar levels were more stable, and he had newfound energy to enjoy his morning walks around the town.

Lunch and dinner became a culinary adventure for Samuel. He experimented with flavorful dishes like grilled chicken with lemon and herbs, or a colorful quinoa salad with roasted vegetables. The cookbook provided clear instructions and nutritional information, making it easy for him to stay on track.

Weeks turned into months, and his visits to the doctor began to yield positive results. His blood sugar levels were improving, and he had even shed some excess weight. He was feeling better than he had in years.

One sunny afternoon, he received a surprise call from his doctor. After reviewing his recent tests, the doctor had some incredible news. His dedication to the diabetic diet had paid off. His diabetes was now well-managed, and he was on the road to recovery.

He couldn't contain his joy. He knew that the "Diabetic Diet Cookbook After 50" had been the key to his success.

With tears of happiness in his eyes, he thanked his daughter for introducing him to the cookbook that had changed his life.

As the seasons changed and the years passed, he continued to savor the flavors of his newfound culinary journey. He walked through the town's hills with a spring in his step, enjoying the beauty of life, all thanks to the power of a healthy diet and the invaluable guidance of the cookbook.

And so, in a small town where Samuel's story became an inspiration to many, the elderly man proved that it's never too late to take control of one's health and savor the sweetness of life with each balanced and delicious meal.

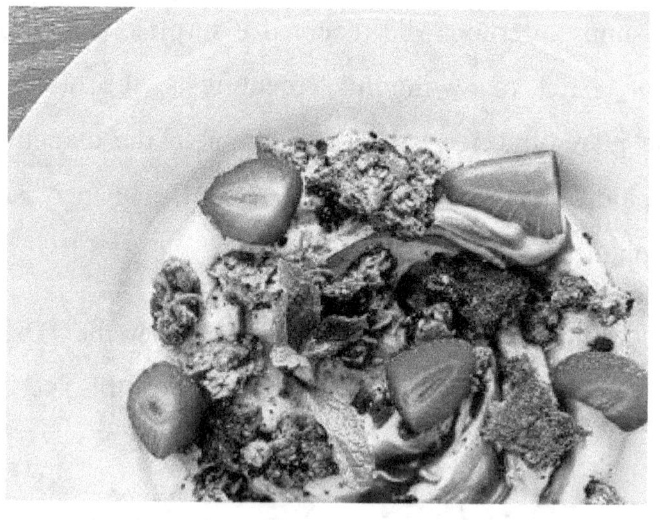

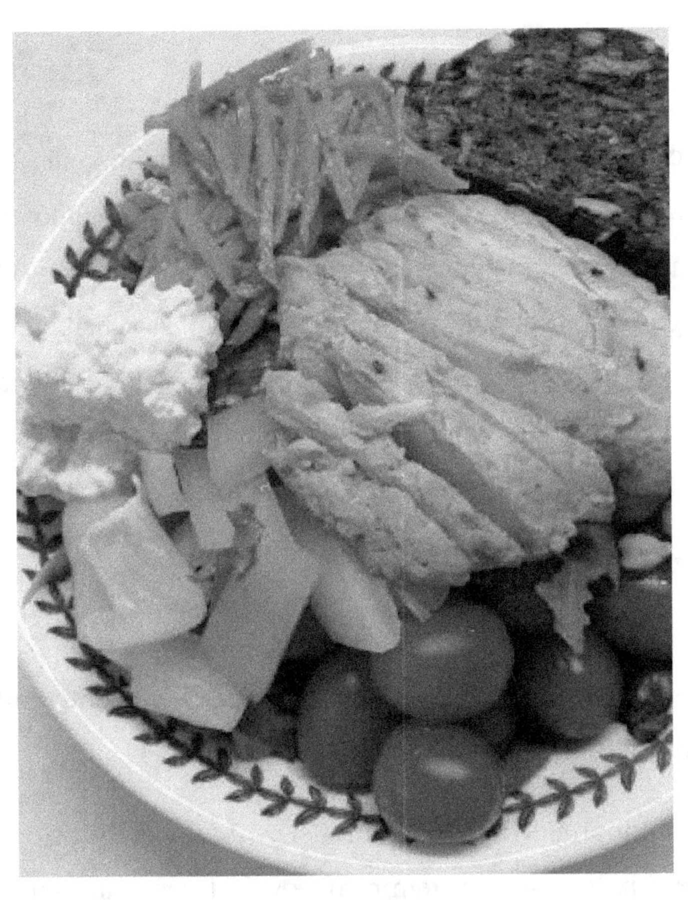

CHAPTER 1

What is Diabetic

Diabetes is a chronic illness that interferes with your body's ability to control blood sugar or glucose. The hormone insulin, which the pancreas produces, aids in the movement of glucose from the circulation into cells, where it may utilized as energy. Glucose is an essential source of energy for the body. High blood sugar levels are the result of either the pancreas not producing enough insulin or the body's inability to use the insulin that is produced.

Types of Diabetics

Type 1, type 2, and gestational diabetes are the three primary subtypes of diabetes.

An autoimmune condition known as type 1 diabetes occurs when the immune system erroneously targets and kills the pancreatic cells that make insulin. Because of this, people with type 1 diabetes produce little to no insulin and need to take insulin throughout their lives. Although it may happen at any age, type 1 diabetes often manifests in childhood or adolescence.

About 90% of instances of diabetes are type 2, making it the most prevalent kind. It happens when the body stops producing enough insulin to maintain normal blood sugar levels or when it develops immunity to the effects of insulin. Poor food, a sedentary lifestyle, obesity, and heredity are among lifestyle variables that are often linked to type 2 diabetes. It usually appears in adults, but because of the growth in juvenile obesity, diagnoses of it in children and adolescents are on the rise.

When the placenta's hormones prevent the body from successfully using insulin during pregnancy, gestational diabetes develops. Although this illness goes away after childbirth, women who have had gestational diabetes are more likely to subsequently acquire type 2 diabetes.

Symptoms of Diabetics

Common symptoms include frequent urination, excessive thirst, unexplained weight loss, increased hunger, fatigue, blurred vision, slow-healing wounds, and frequent infections.

However, some individuals with type 2 diabetes may not experience any symptoms, especially in the early stages of the disease. Depending on the type and severity of the condition, the symptoms can vary.

Preventive Measures for Diabetes

It focuses on lifestyle modifications and early detection. Here are some key strategies to prevent or delay the onset of diabetes:

1. **Healthy Eating**: Adopting a balanced diet rich in fruits, vegetables, whole grains, lean proteins, and healthy fats can help manage weight, regulate blood sugar levels, and reduce the risk of developing diabetes. Incorporating super foods, such as berries, leafy greens, nuts, and seeds, into your meals can provide additional health benefits.

2. **Regular Physical Activity**: Regular exercise, such as brisk walking, jogging, swimming, or cycling, can improve insulin sensitivity, help maintain a healthy weight, and reduce the risk of developing type 2 diabetes. Aim for strength training twice a week and at least 150 minutes of moderate-intensity aerobic activity per week.

3. Weight Management: Maintaining a healthy weight or losing excess weight if overweight or obese is crucial in preventing diabetes. Excess body fat, especially around the abdomen, increases insulin resistance and the risk of developing type 2 diabetes.

4. Stress Reduction: Chronic stress can contribute to the development of diabetes by increasing blood sugar levels and promoting unhealthy behaviors like overeating or lack of physical activity. Practicing stress reduction techniques such as mindfulness meditation, deep breathing exercises, yoga, and aromatherapy can help manage stress levels and reduce the risk of diabetes.

5. Limiting Alcohol Consumption: Excessive alcohol consumption can lead to weight gain, increase blood pressure and triglyceride levels, and impair insulin sensitivity. It is advised to keep alcohol consumption to moderate levels (one drink for women and two for men per day).

6. Avoiding Tobacco Use: Smoking increases the risk of developing type 2 diabetes and other chronic diseases.

Quitting smoking or avoiding tobacco use altogether can significantly reduce the risk of diabetes and improve overall health.

7. Regular medical check-ups: Regular check-ups with your healthcare provider are essential for the early detection and management of diabetes. Routine screenings, including blood glucose tests, can help identify pre diabetes or diabetes in its early stages, when lifestyle modifications may be most effective.

By incorporating these preventive measures into your daily life, you can reduce your risk of developing diabetes and improve your overall health and well-being. It is important to remember that everyone's risk factors and circumstances are unique, so consulting with a healthcare professional is crucial in developing a personalized prevention plan. Taking proactive steps towards a healthier future is the key to preventing diabetes and living a fulfilling life.

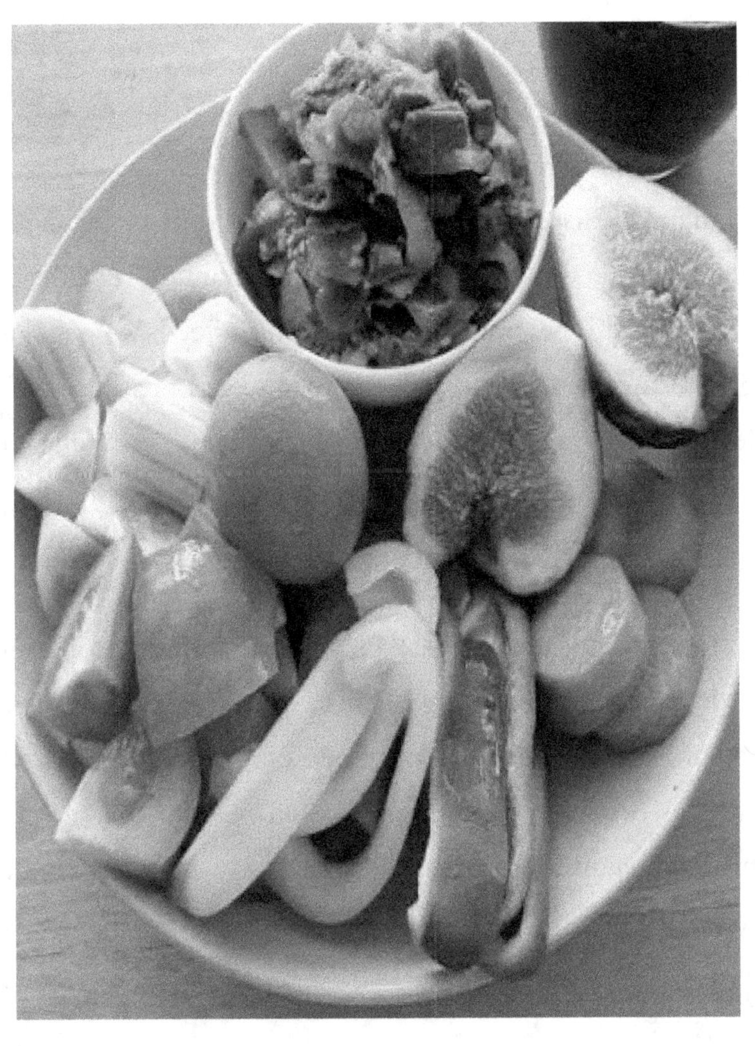

CHAPTER 2

How to Manage Diabetic Diet

A diabetic disease diet plays a crucial role in managing blood sugar levels and achieving optimum health for individuals. The primary goal of this diet is to regulate blood sugar levels and prevent spikes or drops in glucose levels. Here are some foods to eat and avoid on a diabetic disease diet:

Foods to Eat:

1. Fruits and Vegetables: Incorporate a variety of fruits and vegetables into your diet, as they are rich in fiber, vitamins, and minerals. Opt for low-glycemic index fruits such as berries, cherries, apples, and pears. Leafy greens, broccoli, cauliflower, and bell peppers are excellent choices for vegetables.

2. Whole Grains: Choose whole grains over refined grains to ensure a steady release of glucose into the bloodstream. This includes brown rice, quinoa, whole wheat bread, oats, and barley. These grains are high in fiber, which helps regulate blood sugar levels and promotes satiety.

3. Lean Proteins: Include lean protein sources in your meals to help stabilize blood sugar levels and promote feelings of fullness. Good options include skinless chicken or turkey breast, fish (such as salmon or tuna), tofu, legumes (such as lentils or chickpeas), and low-fat dairy products.

4. Healthy Fats: Include healthy fats in your diet, such as avocados, nuts, seeds, and olive oil. These fats may increase insulin sensitivity and support cardiovascular health.

5. Low-Fat Dairy: Choose low-fat or non-fat dairy products like milk, yogurt, and cheese. These provide essential nutrients like calcium and protein without adding excessive saturated fats.

6. Water: Drink a lot of water to stay hydrated. Water has no calories or sugar and can help control appetite and maintain overall health.

Foods to Avoid or Limit:

1. Sugary Foods and Beverages: Avoid or limit foods and drinks that are high in added sugars, such as soda, fruit juices, candy, pastries, and desserts. These can cause rapid spikes in blood sugar levels.

2. Refined Grains: Minimize the consumption of refined grains like white bread, white rice, and pasta. These grains have been processed and stripped of their fiber content, leading to a quicker release of glucose into the bloodstream.

3. Trans Fats and Saturated Fats: Limit the intake of trans fats and saturated fats found in fried foods, processed snacks, high-fat dairy products, and fatty cuts of meat. These fats can increase the risk of heart disease and worsen insulin resistance.

4. High-Sodium Foods: Reduce the consumption of high-sodium foods like processed meats, canned soups, and packaged snacks. Opt for low-sodium alternatives or prepare meals at home using fresh ingredients.

5. Sweetened Beverages: Avoid sugary drinks like soda, sweetened teas, energy drinks, and sports drinks. These beverages can cause a rapid rise in blood sugar levels and contribute to weight gain.

6. Alcohol: Limit alcohol consumption, as it can interfere with blood sugar control and may cause hypoglycemia (low blood sugar) if consumed excessively.

Benefit of Diabetic Disease Diet

Following a diabetic disease diet can provide several core benefits for seniors after 50:

1. Blood Sugar Control: A diabetic disease diet focuses on regulating blood sugar levels, which is crucial for individuals with diabetes. By following this diet, seniors can better manage their blood sugar levels and prevent spikes or drops in glucose levels. This may lower the risk of diabetic complications such as heart disease, renal disease, and nerve damage.

2. Weight Management: A diabetic disease diet emphasizes whole foods that are low in calories and high in nutrients.

This can help seniors maintain a healthy weight or lose excess weight. Maintaining a healthy weight can also reduce the risk of other chronic conditions, such as high blood pressure and arthritis.

3. Heart Health: A diabetic disease diet promotes heart health by limiting the intake of saturated and trans fats, which can increase the risk of heart disease. Instead, it encourages the consumption of healthy fats found in foods like avocados, nuts, and olive oil. By following this diet, seniors can improve their cholesterol levels, reduce inflammation, and lower their risk of heart disease.

4. Nutrient Intake: A diabetic disease diet encourages the consumption of a variety of fruits, vegetables, whole grains, lean proteins, and low-fat dairy products. These foods are good sources of fiber, vitamins, and minerals—all necessary nutrients. Incorporating these foods into their diet can ensure support for their overall health and well-being.

5. Energy Levels: Following a diabetic disease diet can help seniors maintain stable energy levels throughout the day.

By choosing foods that have a low glycemic index (such as whole grains and vegetables), seniors can avoid rapid spikes and drops in blood sugar levels that can lead to fatigue and energy crashes.

6. Digestive Health: The high fiber content in a diabetic disease diet can promote healthy digestion and prevent constipation. Fiber helps regulate bowel movements and keeps the digestive system functioning. Seniors can benefit from improved digestive health and a reduced risk of gastrointestinal issues by following this diet.

Overall, following a diabetic disease diet can provide seniors after 50 with better blood sugar control, weight management, heart health, improved nutrient intake, stable energy levels, and enhanced digestive health. Seniors need to work with a healthcare professional or registered dietitian to create an individualized meal plan that meets their specific needs and preferences. Regular monitoring of blood sugar levels is also essential to assess the effectiveness of the diet and make any necessary adjustments.

CHAPTER 3

The Power of a Balanced Diet

To follow a diabetic disease diet after 50, focus on managing blood sugar levels and preventing complications associated with diabetes. Here are some steps to help you navigate this dietary journey:

1. Understand the Diabetic Disease After 50:

- Educate yourself about the impact of diabetes on individuals over the age of 50.
- Recognize the importance of a healthy diet.
- Learn about the potential complications that can arise if the proper diet is not adopted.

2. Embrace a Comprehensive Approach:

- Adopt principles of a diabetic diet, such as portion control, carbohydrate management, and mindful eating.
- Work with a healthcare professional or registered dietitian to create a personalized meal plan that suits your needs.

- Use practical meal planning and preparation to make healthy eating more manageable.

3. Build Your Shopping List:

- Include a variety of nutrient-rich foods in your diabetic diet.
- Focus on foods low in added sugars, saturated fats, and sodium.
- Incorporate whole grains, lean proteins, fruits, vegetables, and healthy fats into your shopping list.

4. Cook for Wellness:

- Explore simple and flavorful recipes that align with your diabetic diet.
- Prioritize balanced meals that include a mix of carbohydrates, proteins, and fats.
- Experiment with different flavors and adapt recipes to suit your preferences.

5. Overcome Challenges and Stay Motivated:

- Be prepared for common obstacles, such as dining out or managing cravings.
- Seek support from friends, family, or support groups to stay motivated.
- Celebrate small victories and remind yourself of the positive impact a healthy diet can have on your overall well-being.

Comprehensive List of Essential Ingredients

Here are 20 healthy shopping ingredients or items that can be included in a diabetic disease diet:

1. Whole grains: brown rice, quinoa, whole wheat bread, and whole grain pasta.

2. Lean proteins: skinless chicken breast, turkey breast, fish (such as salmon or trout), tofu, and eggs.

3. Low-fat dairy products: Greek yogurt, skim milk, and low-fat cheese.

4. Fresh fruits: berries (such as strawberries, blueberries, and raspberries), apples, oranges, and grapes.

5. Non-starchy vegetables: leafy greens (spinach, kale, and lettuce), broccoli, cauliflower, bell peppers, and zucchini.

6. Legumes: lentils, chickpeas, black beans, and kidney beans.

7. Healthy fats: avocado, olive oil, nuts (almonds and walnuts), and seeds (flaxseeds and chia seeds).

8. Herbs and spices: garlic, ginger, turmeric, cinnamon, and oregano.

9. Low-sodium condiments: mustard, vinegar, salsa, and hot sauce.

10. Sugar alternatives: Stevia or monk fruit sweeteners for reducing added sugar intake.

11. Unsweetened beverages: water, herbal tea, and unsweetened almond or coconut milk.

12. Canned goods: low-sodium canned vegetables, tuna or salmon (packed in water), and no-added-sugar canned fruits.

13. Nut butter: natural peanut butter or almond butter without added sugars or hydrogenated oils.

14. Whole-grain snacks: Whole-grain crackers or popcorn.

15. Frozen vegetables: convenient options for adding vegetables to meals.

16. Dark chocolate: In moderation, dark chocolate with a high cocoa content can be a healthier option.

17. Vinegar: balsamic vinegar or apple cider vinegar for salad dressings or marinades.

18. Herbal supplements: Consult a healthcare professional for recommended supplements such as cinnamon or alpha-lipoic acid.

19. Canned or dried herbs: basil, parsley, cilantro, and thyme for adding flavor to meals without sodium

20. High-fiber cereals: Look for low-added sugars and high-fiber content.

Risk Factor

If the right diet is not adopted for diabetes after the age of 50, several complications can arise. These complications can include:

1. Cardiovascular disease: Diabetes increases the risk of heart disease, including coronary artery disease, heart attacks, and strokes. Poor diet choices can further elevate this risk.

2. High blood pressure: Uncontrolled diabetes can lead to high blood pressure and increase the risk of heart disease, stroke, and kidney problems.

3. Kidney disease: Diabetes is among the causes of kidney disease. Lack of proper diet management and high blood sugar levels can damage the kidneys over time, leading to kidney failure.

4. Diabetic retinopathy: This condition affects the eyes and can lead to vision loss or blindness. Poorly controlled blood sugar levels can accelerate the progression of diabetic retinopathy.

5. Neuropathy: Nerve damage is a common complication of diabetes. It can cause pain, tingling, or numbness in the hands, feet, or other parts of the body.

6. Foot problems: Diabetes can impair blood flow and nerve function in the feet, increasing the risk of infections, ulcers, and even amputations if left untreated.

7. Skin conditions: High blood sugar levels can contribute to skin problems such as infections, slow wound healing, and dryness.

8. Gastroparesis: This condition affects the digestive system and causes delayed emptying of the stomach. It can lead to symptoms like nausea, vomiting, bloating, and a poor appetite.

9. Increased susceptibility to infections: High blood sugar levels can weaken the immune system, making individuals with diabetes more prone to infections, especially urinary tract infections and skin infections.

10. Mental health issues: Diabetes can have a significant impact on mental health, leading to increased rates of depression, anxiety, and stress if not managed properly.

It is crucial for individuals with diabetes after the age of 50 to adopt a healthy diet and lifestyle to minimize the risk of these complications. Regular exercise, medication management, and regular check-ups with healthcare professionals are essential for overall diabetes management.

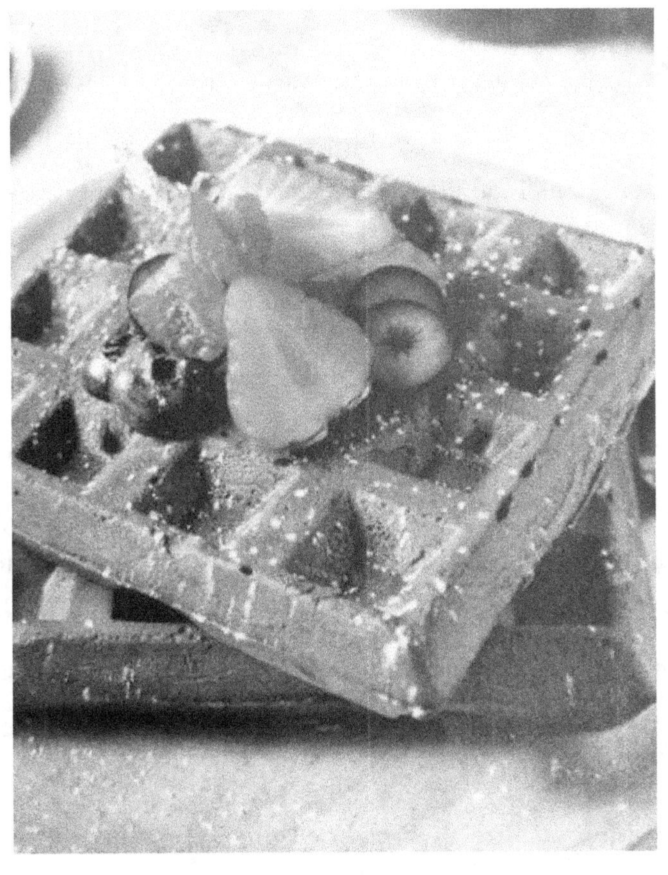

CHAPTER 4

The Plate Method for Balanced Meals

The plate method is a simple and effective way to create balanced meals that support blood sugar control. Imagine your plate divided into three sections: one-half for non-starchy vegetables, one-quarter for lean proteins, and one-quarter for whole grains or starchy vegetables. By following this method, you ensure that your meals are filled with essential nutrients while keeping carbohydrates in check.

Portion Sizes for Older Adults

As we age, our nutritional needs may change, and portion sizes become even more important. Older adults should focus on consuming adequate protein to support muscle health and limit carbohydrate intake to manage blood sugar levels. A general guideline is to have a palm-sized portion of protein, a fist-sized portion of non-starchy vegetables, and a cupped hand-sized portion of whole grains or starchy vegetables.

Meal Plans Samples

Creating meal plans can be overwhelming, especially if you have specific dietary preferences. To make it easier, we have provided sample meal plans for different dietary preferences, including vegetarian, vegan, and gluten-free options. These meal plans include a variety of nutrient-dense foods to keep you satisfied and support your blood sugar control goals.

7-Day Diabetic Disease Meal Plan Sample:

Day 1

Breakfast: Eggs scrambled with tomatoes and spinach

Snack: Greek yogurt with berries

Lunch: Mixed greens salad with grilled chicken and vinaigrette

Snack: Cucumber and carrot sticks with hummus

Dinner: Baked salmon with quinoa and steamed broccoli

Dessert: Sugar-free gelatin

Day 2

Breakfast oatmeal with banana slices and a dash of cinnamon

Snack: Almonds

Lunch: Turkey and avocado whole wheat wrap with a side of mixed greens

Snack: Celery sticks with peanut butter

Dinner: Brown rice with veggies and Stir-fried tofu

Dessert: Sugar-free pudding

Day 3

Breakfast: Greek yogurt parfait with granola and strawberries

Snack: Sliced apples with a light cheese

Lunch: Side salad with lentil soup

Snack: Cherry tomatoes with balsamic vinegar

Dinner: Grilled shrimp with asparagus and quinoa

Dessert: Mixed berries with a dollop of whipped cream (sugar-free)

Day 4

Breakfast: Banana slices with whole-grain toast with almond butter

Snack: Cottage cheese with pineapple chunks

Lunch: Chickpea, cucumber, and feta cheese in a quinoa salad

Snack: Mixed nuts

Dinner: Sweet potato and green beans with baked chicken breast

Dessert: Sugar-free dark chocolate

Day 5

Breakfast: Omelet with a side of whole grain toast eith veggie omelet

Snack: Sliced pears with a small handful of walnuts

Lunch: Brown rice with turkey and vegetable stir-fry

Snack: Celery sticks with cream cheese

Dinner: Baked cod with steamed asparagus and quinoa

Dessert: Sugar-free ice cream or sorbet

Day 6

Breakfast: Spinach, banana, Greek yogurt, and almond milk smoothie

Snack: Sliced cucumbers with tzatziki sauce

 Lunch: Chicken breast filled with spinach and feta served with a side salad

Snack: Hard-boiled eggs

Dinner: Beef and vegetable kebabs with brown rice

Dessert: Sliced peaches with a sprinkle of cinnam

Day 7

Breakfast: Cottage cheese with mixed berries and a drizzle of honey

Snack: Baby carrots with hummus

Lunch: Quinoa and black bean salad with a lime vinaigrette

Snack: Mixed nuts

Dinner: Grilled turkey burger with a lettuce wrap and a side of roasted Brussels sprouts

Dessert: Sugar-free fruit salad

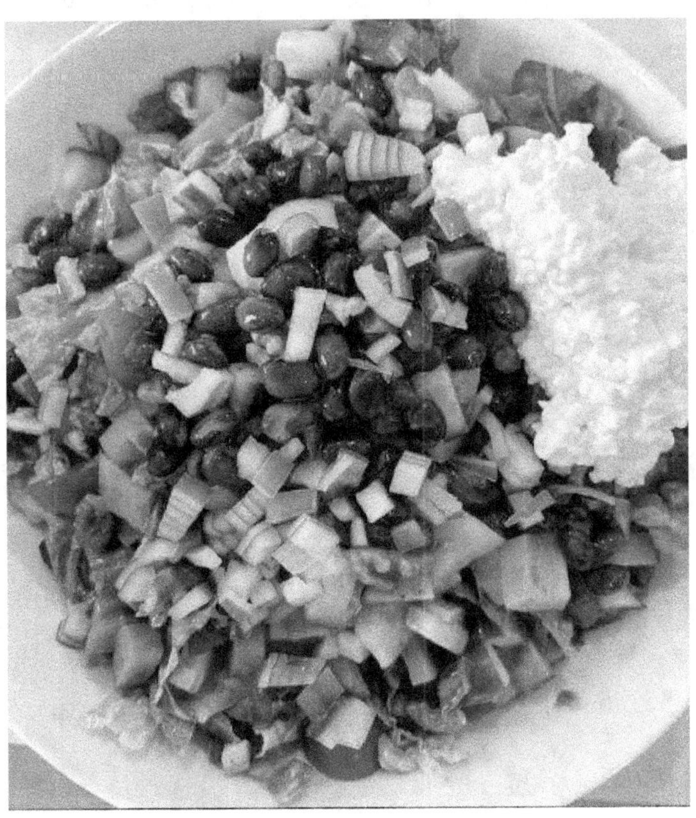

Chapter 5

Recipe

In this chapter we will dive into a collection of diabetic-friendly recipes that are not only delicious but also support blood sugar control. From breakfast to dinner and even snacks, these recipes will provide you with balanced, flavorful, and satisfying meals. Each recipe comes with clear instructions, nutritional information, and tips for customization, so you can tailor them to your preferences. Let's get cooking!

Breakfast Recipes

1. Veggie Omelet:

Ingredients:

- 2 eggs

- 1/4 cup bell peppers, diced

- 1/4 cup spinach, chopped

- 1/4 cup mushrooms, sliced

- 1 tablespoon low-fat cheese

- Salt and pepper to taste

Nutritional Value:

- Calories: 200

- Carbohydrates: 8g

- Protein: 15g

- Fat: 12g

- Fiber: 3g

Preparation:

1. In a bowl, whisk the eggs together with salt and pepper.

2. Spray cooking spray onto a non-stick skillet and heat it up over medium heat.

3. Add the bell peppers, spinach, and mushrooms to the skillet and cook until softened.

4. Pour the whisked eggs over the vegetables and cook until set.

5. Sprinkle the omelet with low-fat cheese and fold in half.

6. Cook for another minute until the cheese is melted.

7. Serve hot.

Cooking Time: 10 minutes

2. Overnight Chia Pudding:

Ingredients:

- 2 tablespoons chia seeds

- 1/2 cup unsweetened almond milk

- 1/4 teaspoon vanilla extract

- Fresh berries or nuts for topping

Nutritional Value:

- Calories: 150

- Carbohydrates: 10g

- Protein: 5g

- Fat: 9g

- Fiber: 8g

Preparation:

1. In a jar or bowl, mix the chia seeds, almond milk, and vanilla extract.

2. Stir well to combine and make sure there are no clumps of chia seeds.

3. Refrigerate overnight while the jar is covered.

4. In the morning, give the chia pudding a stir and top it with fresh berries or nuts.

5. Enjoy chilled.

Cooking Time: Overnight

3. Whole Grain Pancakes:

Ingredients:

- 1 cup whole wheat flour

- 1 tablespoon baking powder

- 1/4 teaspoon salt

- 1 cup unsweetened almond milk

- 1 tablespoon honey or sugar substitute

- Fresh fruit or sugar-free syrup for topping

Nutritional Value:

- Calories: 200

- Carbohydrates: 40g

- Protein: 8g

- Fat: 2g

- Fiber: 6g

Preparation:

1. In a bowl, whisk together the whole wheat flour, baking powder, and salt.

2. In a separate bowl, mix the almond milk and honey (or sugar substitute).

3. Mix the dry ingredients until it incorporated

4. Spray cooking spray onto a nonstick skillet and heat it over medium heat.

5. Pour 1/4 cup of the pancake batter onto the skillet and cook until bubbles form on the surface.

6. Flip the pancake and cook for another minute until golden brown.

7. Repeat with the remaining batter.

8. Serve the pancakes with fresh fruit or sugar-free syrup.

Cooking Time: 15 minutes

4. Greek Yogurt Parfait:

Ingredients:

- 1/2 cup low-fat Greek yogurt

- 1/4 cup fresh berries

- 2 tablespoons granola

Nutritional Value:

- Calories: 150

- Carbohydrates: 20g

- Protein: 10g

- Fat: 3g

- Fiber: 4g

Preparation:

1. In a glass or bowl, layer the Greek yogurt, fresh berries, and granola.

2. Repeat until all the ingredients are finished.

3. Serve chilled.

Cooking Time: 5 minutes

5. Avocado Toast:

Ingredients:

- 1 slice whole grain bread

- 1/4 avocado, mashed

- 2 slices tomato

- 1 poached egg (optional)

- Salt and pepper to taste

Nutritional Value:

- Calories: 200

- Carbohydrates: 20g

- Protein: 10g

- Fat: 10g

- Fiber: 6g

Preparation:

1. Toast the slice of whole grain bread.

2. Spread the mashed avocado on top of the toast.

3. Place the tomato slices on top of the avocado.

4. Optional: Top with a poached egg.

5. Season with salt and pepper.

6. Serve immediately.

Cooking Time: 10 minutes

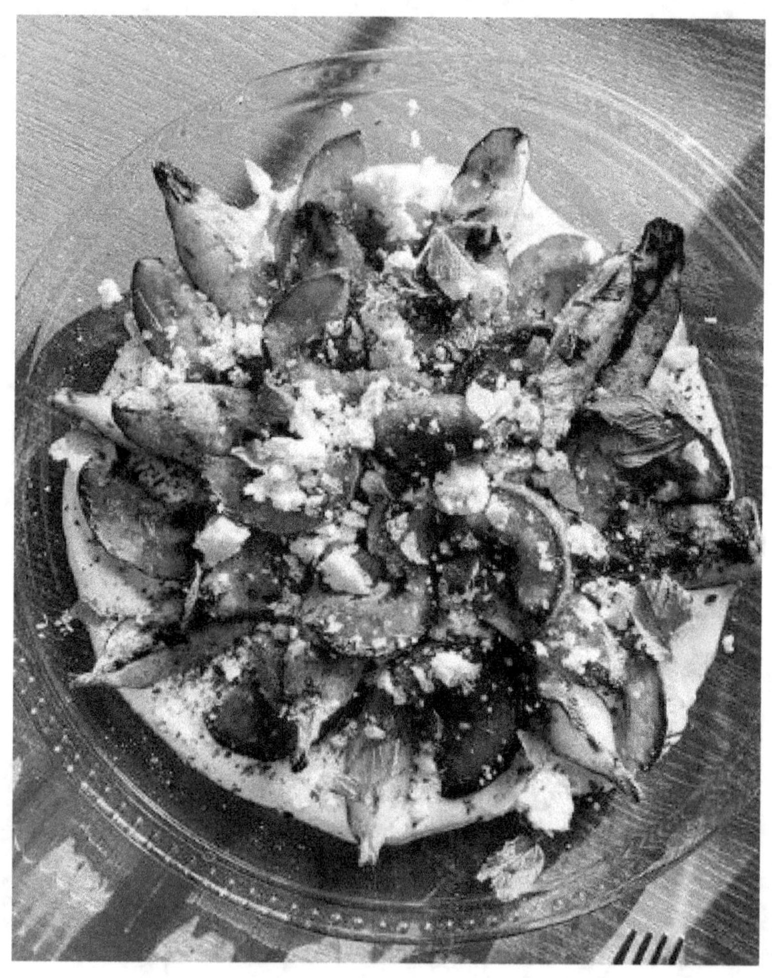

Lunch Recipe

1. Grilled Chicken Salad:

Ingredients:

- 4 oz grilled chicken breast, sliced

- 2 cups mixed salad greens

- 1/4 cup cherry tomatoes, halved

- 1/4 cup cucumber, sliced

- 1/4 cup bell peppers, diced

- 1 tablespoon olive oil

- 1 tablespoon balsamic vinegar

- Salt and pepper to taste

Nutritional Value:

- Calories: 250

- Carbohydrates: 10g

- Protein: 30g

- Fat: 10g

- Fiber: 4g

Preparation:

1. In a bowl, combine the mixed salad greens, cherry tomatoes, cucumber, and bell peppers.

2. Drizzle the olive oil and balsamic vinegar over the salad.

3. Season with salt and pepper.

4. Top the salad with sliced grilled chicken breast.

5. Toss gently to combine.

6. Serve chilled.

Cooking Time: 15 minutes

2. Turkey and Avocado Wrap:

Ingredients:

- 4 oz turkey breast, sliced

- 1/4 avocado, sliced

- 1 whole wheat tortilla

- 1/4 cup spinach leaves

- 1 tablespoon mustard or low-fat mayo (optional)

Nutritional Value:

- Calories: 300

- Carbohydrates: 25g

- Protein: 25g

- Fat: 10g

- Fiber: 6g

Preparation:

1. Lay the whole wheat tortilla flat on a clean surface.

2. Spread mustard or low-fat mayo (if desired) on the tortilla.

3. Layer the spinach leaves, turkey breast slices, and avocado slices on top of the tortilla.

4. Roll up the tortilla tightly.

5. Slice the wrap in half.

6. Serve at room temperature.

Cooking Time: 5 minutes

3. Salmon and Quinoa Salad:

Ingredients:

- 4 oz grilled salmon fillet

- 1/2 cup cooked quinoa

- 1 cup mixed salad greens

- 1/4 cup cherry tomatoes, halved

- 1/4 cup cucumber, sliced

- 1 tablespoon lemon juice

- Salt and pepper to taste

Nutritional Value:

- Calories: 350

- Carbohydrates: 25g

- Protein: 30g

- Fat: 15g

- Fiber: 4g

Preparation:

1. In a bowl, combine the mixed salad greens, cherry tomatoes, and cucumber.

2. Squeeze lemon juice over the salad.

3. Season with salt and pepper.

4. Top the salad with grilled salmon fillet and cooked quinoa.

5. Toss gently to combine.

6. Serve chilled.

Cooking Time: 20 minutes

4. Veggie Stir-Fry with Tofu:

Ingredients:

- 4 oz tofu, cubed

- 1 cup mixed vegetablessliced

- 1 tablespoon low-sodium soy sauce

- 1 tablespoon sesame oil

- 1/4 teaspoon garlic powder

- 1/4 teaspoon ginger powder

- Salt and pepper to taste

Nutritional Value:

- Calories: 200

- Carbohydrates: 15g

- Protein: 15g

- Fat: 10g

- Fiber: 6g

Preparation:

1. Heat the sesame oil in a non-stick skillet over medium heat.

2. Add the tofu cubes to the skillet and cook until lightly browned.

3. Add the mixed vegetables to the skillet and stir-fry until tender.

4. In a small bowl, whisk together the low-sodium soy sauce, garlic powder, and ginger powder.

5. Pour the sauce over the tofu and vegetables in the skillet.

6. Season with salt and pepper.

7. Stir-fry for an additional 2-3 minutes.

8. Serve hot.

Cooking Time: 15 minutes

5. Quinoa Stuffed Bell Peppers:

Ingredients:

- 2 bell peppers, halved and seeded

- 1 cup cooked quinoa

- 1/4 cup black beans, rinsed and drained

- 1/4 cup corn kernels

- 1/4 cup diced tomatoes

- 1/4 cup shredded low-fat cheese

- 1/4 teaspoon cumin

- Salt and pepper to taste

Nutritional Value:

- Calories: 250

- Carbohydrates: 30g

- Protein: 10g

- Fat: 5g

- Fiber: 6g

Preparation:

1. Preheat the oven to 375°F (190°C).

2. In a bowl, combine the cooked quinoa, black beans, corn kernels, diced tomatoes, shredded cheese, cumin, salt, and pepper.

3. Stuff the bell pepper halves with the quinoa mixture.

4. Arrange the stuffed bell peppers on a baking pan.

5. Bake in the preheated oven for 20-25 minutes or until the peppers are tender and the cheese is melted.

6. Serve hot.

Cooking Time: 30 minutes

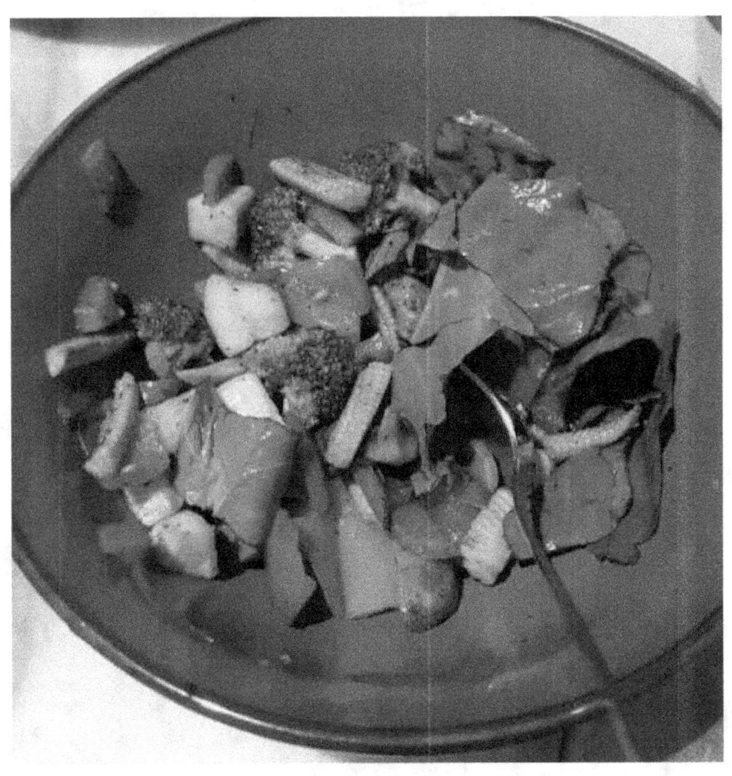

Dinner Recipe

1. Greek Salad with Chicken:

Ingredients:

- 4 oz grilled chicken breast, sliced

- 2 cups mixed salad greens

- 1/4 cup cherry tomatoes, halved

- 1/4 cup cucumber, sliced

- 1/4 cup Kalamata olives, pitted

- 1/4 cup feta cheese, crumbled

- 1 tablespoon olive oil

- 1 tablespoon lemon juice

- Salt and pepper to taste

Nutritional Value:

- Calories: 300

- Carbohydrates: 10g

- Protein: 30g

- Fat: 15g

- Fiber: 4g

Preparation:

1. In a bowl, combine the mixed salad greens, cherry tomatoes, cucumber, Kalamata olives, and feta cheese.

2. Over the salad, drizzle some olive oil and lemon juice.

3. Season with salt and pepper.

4. Top the salad with sliced grilled chicken breast.

5. Toss gently to combine.

6. Serve chilled.

Cooking Time: 15 minutes

2. Lentil Soup:

Ingredients:

- 1/2 cup lentils, rinsed and drained

- 1/4 cup diced onion

- 1/4 cup diced carrots

- 1/4 cup diced celery

- 2 cups low-sodium vegetable broth

- 1/2 teaspoon cumin

- 1/4 teaspoon paprika

- Salt and pepper to taste

Nutritional Value:

- Calories: 200

- Carbohydrates: 30g

- Protein: 15g

- Fat: 1g

- Fiber: 10g

Preparation:

1. In a pot, combine the lentils, diced onion, diced carrots, diced celery, vegetable broth, cumin, paprika, salt, and pepper.

2. Over medium-high heat, bring the combination to a boil.

3. Reduce the heat to low and simmer for 20-25 minutes or until the lentils are tender.

4. Serve hot.

Cooking Time: 30 minutes

3. Tuna Salad Lettuce Wraps:

Ingredients:

- 4 oz canned tuna in water, drained

- 1/4 cup diced celery

- 1/4 cup diced red onion

- 1 tablespoon low-fat Greek yogurt

- 1 tablespoon lemon juice

- Salt and pepper to taste

- Lettuce leaves for wrapping

Nutritional Value:

- Calories: 150

- Carbohydrates: 5g

- Protein: 20g

- Fat: 5g

- Fiber: 2g

Preparation:

1. In a bowl, combine the canned tuna, diced celery, diced red onion, Greek yogurt, lemon juice, salt, and pepper.

2. Stir well to combine.

3. Place a spoon of tuna salad on each lettuce leaf.

4. In order to make wraps, roll the lettuce leaves.

5. Serve chilled.

Cooking Time: 10 minutes

4. Caprese Salad:

Ingredients:

- 1 large tomato, sliced

- 1/4 cup fresh mozzarella cheese, sliced

- 1/4 cup fresh basil leaves

- 1 tablespoon balsamic vinegar

- 1 tablespoon olive oil

- Salt and pepper to taste

Nutritional Value:

- Calories: 200

- Carbohydrates: 10g

- Protein: 8g

- Fat: 15g

- Fiber: 2g

Preparation:

1. Place the tomato slices on a plate.

2. Top each tomato slice with a slice of fresh mozzarella cheese.

3. Place a fresh basil leaf on top of each cheese slice.

4. Over the salad, drizzle the olive oil and balsamic vinegar..

5. Season with salt and pepper.

6. Serve at room temperature.

Cooking Time: 5 minutes

5. Chicken and Vegetable Stir-Fry:

Ingredients:

- 4 oz chicken breast, sliced

- 1 cup mixed vegetables sliced

- 1 tablespoon low-sodium soy sauce

- 1 tablespoon olive oil

- 1/4 teaspoon garlic powder

- 1/4 teaspoon ginger powder

- Salt and pepper to taste

Nutritional Value:

- Calories: 250

- Carbohydrates: 15g

- Protein: 25g

- Fat: 10g

- Fiber: 6g

Preparation:

1. In a nonstick skillet, warm the olive oil over medium heat.

2. Add the chicken breast slices to the skillet and cook until lightly browned.

3. Add the mixed vegetables to the skillet and stir-fry until tender.

4. In a small bowl, whisk together the low-sodium soy sauce, garlic powder, and ginger powder.

5. Pour the sauce over the chicken and vegetables in the skillet.

6. Season with salt and pepper.

7. Stir-fry for an additional 2-3 minutes.

8. Serve hot.

Cooking Time: 15 minutes

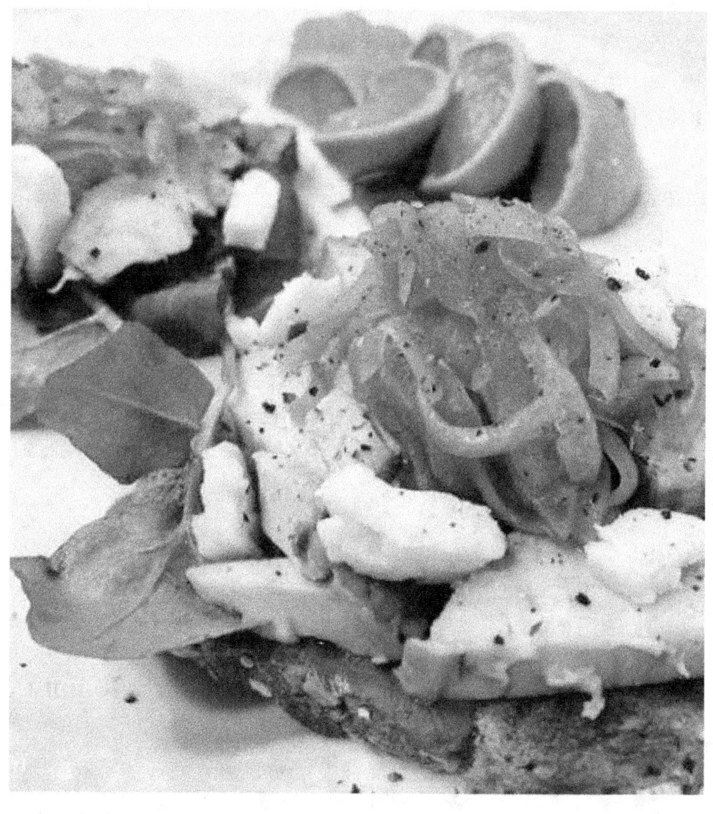

1. Veggie and Hummus Platter:

Ingredients:

- 1 cup sliced cucumber

- 1 cup sliced bell peppers

- 1 cup cherry tomatoes

- 1 cup baby carrots

Preparation:

1. Arrange the sliced cucumber, bell peppers, cherry tomatoes, and baby carrots on a platter.

2. Serve with a side of hummus for dipping.

2. Greek Yogurt Parfait:

Ingredients:

- 1/2 cup plain Greek yogurt

- 1/4 cup mixed berries (such as strawberries, blueberries, and raspberries)

- 1 tablespoon chopped nuts

- 1 teaspoon honey (optional)

Nutritional Value:

- Calories: 150

- Carbohydrates: 15g

- Protein: 15g

- Fat: 5g

- Fiber: 3g

Preparation:

1. In a glass or bowl, layer the Greek yogurt, mixed berries, and chopped nuts.

2. Drizzle with honey if desired.

3. Serve chilled.

3. Caprese Skewers:

Ingredients:

- 8 cherry tomatoes

- 8 small fresh mozzarella balls

- 8 fresh basil leaves

- Balsamic glaze for drizzling

Nutritional Value:

- Calories: 100

- Carbohydrates: 4g

- Protein: 6g

- Fat: 7g

- Fiber: 0g

Preparation:

1. Thread a cherry tomato, fresh mozzarella ball, and fresh basil leaf onto a skewer.

2. Repeat with the remaining ingredients to make a total of 8 skewers.

3. Drizzle with balsamic glaze.

4. Serve at room temperature.

4. Baked Zucchini Fries:

Ingredients:

- 2 medium zucchini, cut into fries

- 1/4 cup grated Parmesan cheese

- 1/4 cup almond flour

- 1/2 teaspoon garlic powder

- Salt and pepper to taste

- Olive oil cooking spray

Nutritional Value:

- Calories: 100

- Carbohydrates: 8g

- Protein: 6g

- Fat: 5g

- Fiber: 3g

Preparation:

1. Preheat the oven to 425°F (220°C).

2. In a bowl, combine the grated Parmesan cheese, almond flour, garlic powder, salt, and pepper.

3. Dip each zucchini fry into the Parmesan mixture, pressing it onto the zucchini to coat evenly.

4. Place the coated zucchini fries on a baking sheet lined with parchment paper.

5. Spray the zucchini fries with olive oil cooking spray.

6. Bake in the preheated oven for 15-20 minutes or until golden brown and crispy.

7. Serve hot.

5. Cucumber and Tuna Bites:

Ingredients:

- 1 cucumber, sliced into rounds

- 1 can tuna in water, drained

- 1/4 cup diced red onion

- 1 tablespoon low-fat Greek yogurt

- Salt and pepper to taste

Nutritional Value:

- Calories: 150

- Carbohydrates: 5g

- Protein: 20g

- Fat: 5g

- Fiber: 2g

Preparation:

1. In a bowl, combine the drained tuna, diced red onion, Greek yogurt, salt, and pepper.

2. Stir well to combine.

3. Place a spoonful of the tuna mixture on top of each cucumber round.

4. Serve chilled.

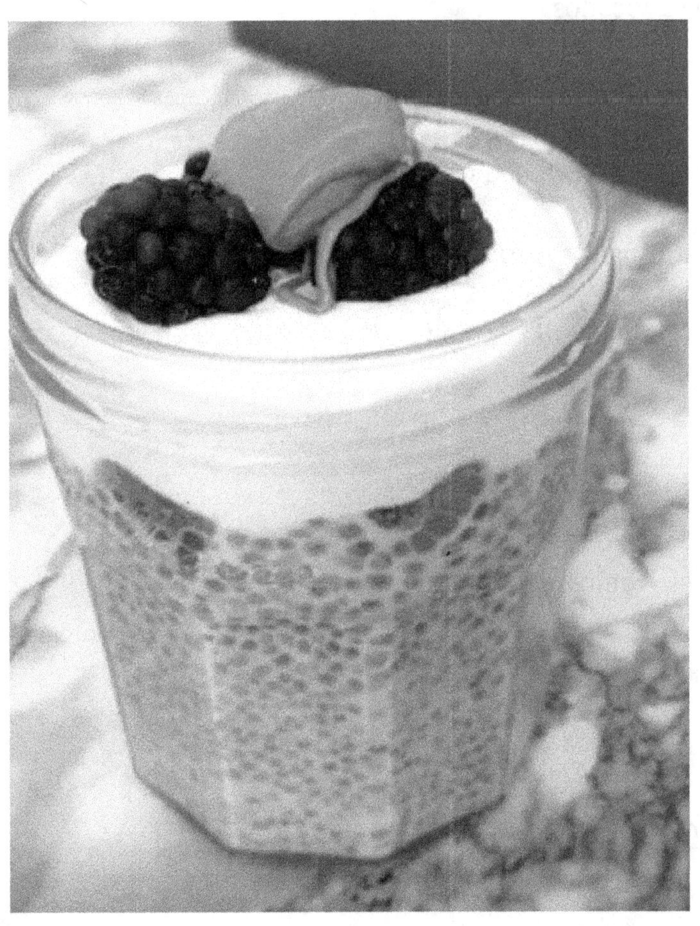

Dessert and sweet treat

1. Sugar-Free Chocolate Avocado Mousse:

Ingredients:

- 2 ripe avocados

- 1/4 cup unsweetened cocoa powder

- 1/4 cup unsweetened almond milk

- 1/4 cup sugar substitute stevia or erythritol

- 1 teaspoon vanilla extract

Nutritional Value:

- Calories: 150

- Carbohydrates: 10g

- Protein: 3g

- Fat: 13g

- Fiber: 7g

Preparation:

1. In a blender or food processor, combine the avocados, cocoa powder, almond milk, sugar substitute, and vanilla extract.

2. Blend until smooth and creamy.

3. Pour the mousse in to glasses.

4. Put in fridge for at least 1 hour before serving.

5. Serve chilled.

2. Berry Chia Pudding:

Ingredients:

- 1/4 cup chia seeds

- 1 cup unsweetened almond milk

- 1/2 cup mixed berries (such as strawberries, blueberries, and raspberries)

- 1 tablespoon sugar substitute stevia or erythritol

Nutritional Value:

- Calories: 100

- Carbohydrates: 10g

- Protein: 4g

- Fat: 5g

- Fiber: 8g

Preparation:

1. Mix the chia seeds and almond milk in a bowl

2. Stir well to combine.

3. Let the mixture sit for 5 minutes, then stir again to break up any clumps.

4. Refrigerate for at least 2 hours or overnight while the bowl is covered.

5. In a separate bowl, mash the mixed berries with a fork.

6. Stir in the sugar substitute.

7. To serve, layer the chia pudding and mashed berries in a glass or bowl.

8. Serve chilled.

3. Peanut Butter Banana Ice Cream:

Ingredients:

- 2 ripe bananas, sliced and frozen

- 2 tablespoons natural peanut butter

- 1 tablespoon unsweetened cocoa powder (optional)

- 1/4 cup chopped peanuts (optional)

Nutritional Value:

- Calories: 200

- Carbohydrates: 25g

- Protein: 5g

- Fat: 10g

- Fiber: 4g

Preparation:

1. In a blender or food processor, combine the frozen banana slices, peanut butter, and cocoa powder (if using).

2. Blend until smooth and creamy.

3. Pour the mixture to in a safe container.

4. Freeze for at least 2 hours or until firm.

5. Scoop the ice cream into serving bowls or cones.

6. Top with chopped peanuts (if desired).

7. Serve frozen.

4. Baked Apple Crisp:

Ingredients:

- 2 medium apples peeled and sliced

- 1/4 cup almond flour

- 1/4 cup rolled oats

- 1/4 cup chopped walnuts

- 2 tablespoons sugar substitute optional

- 1 teaspoon cinnamon

- 2 tablespoons melted coconut oil

Nutritional Value:

- Calories: 150

- Carbohydrates: 20g

- Protein: 3g

- Fat: 8g

- Fiber: 6g

Preparation:

1. Preheat the oven to 375°F (190°C).

2. In a bowl, combine the almond flour, rolled oats, chopped walnuts, sugar substitute, cinnamon, and melted coconut oil.

3. Stir well to combine.

4. Place the sliced apples in a baking dish.

5. Sprinkle the almond flour mixture evenly over the apples.

6. Bake in the preheated oven for 25-30 minutes or until the apples are tender and the topping is golden brown.

7. Serve warm.

5. Lemon Poppy Seed Muffins:

Ingredients:

- 1 cup almond flour

- 1/4 cup coconut flour

- 1/4 cup sugar substitute

- 1 tablespoon poppy seeds

- 1 teaspoon baking powder

- 1/2 teaspoon baking soda

- 1/4 teaspoon salt

- Zest of 1 lemon

- Juice of 1 lemon

- 1/4 cup melted coconut oil

- 3 large eggs

Nutritional Value:

- Calories: 150

- Carbohydrates: 8g

- Protein: 6g

- Fat: 12g

- Fiber: 4g

Preparation:

1. Preheat the oven to 350°F (175°C).

2. In a bowl, combine the almond flour, coconut flour, sugar substitute, poppy seeds, baking powder, baking soda, salt, and lemon zest.

3. In a separate bowl, whisk together the lemon juice, melted coconut oil, and eggs.

4. Combine the wet ingredients with the dry ingredients and stir until well mixed.

5. place paper liners in to muffin cups.

6. Pour the batter evenly among the muffin cups.

7. Bake in the preheated oven for 20-25 minutes or until a toothpick inserted into the center comes out clean.

8. Serving while its cooled.

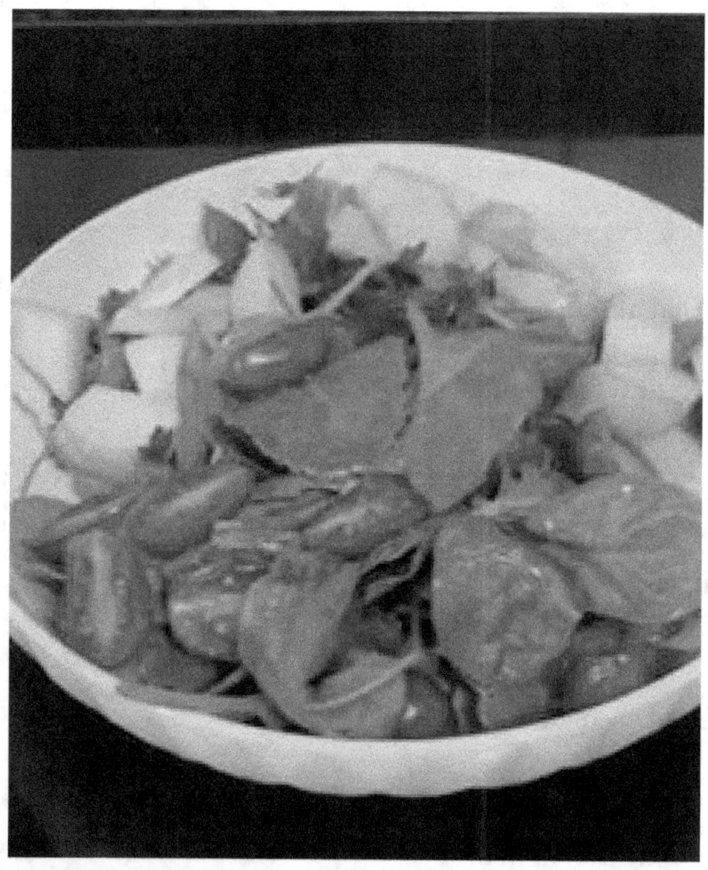

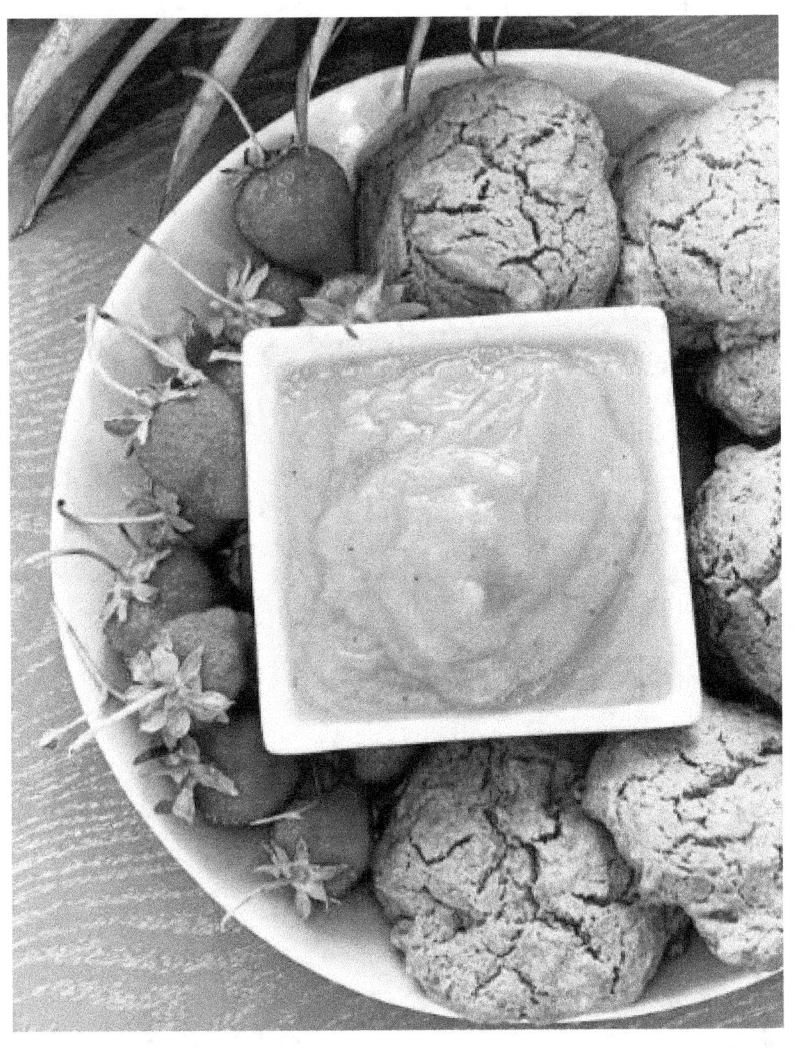

Smoothie and Beverages

1. Green Smoothie:

Ingredients:

- 1 cup spinach

- 1/2 medium avocado

- 1/2 cucumber

- 1/2 cup unsweetened almond milk

- 1 tablespoon chia seeds

- 1 teaspoon sugar substitute

- Juice of 1/2 lemon

Nutritional Value:

- Calories: 100

- Carbohydrates: 10g

- Protein: 4g

- Fat: 6g

- Fiber: 7g

Preparation:

1. In a blender, combine the spinach, avocado, cucumber, almond milk, chia seeds, sugar substitute, and lemon juice.

2. Blend until smooth and creamy.

3. Add ice if desired for a colder smoothie.

4. Pour into a glass and serve chilled.

2. Berry Blast Smoothie:

Ingredients:

- 1 cup mixed berries

- 1/2 cup unsweetened almond milk

- 1/4 cup Greek yogurt

- 1 tablespoon sugar substitute

- 1 tablespoon flaxseed meal

Nutritional Value:

- Calories: 120

- Carbohydrates: 15g

- Protein: 5g

- Fat: 4g

- Fiber: 8g

Preparation:

1. In a blender, combine the mixed berries, almond milk, Greek yogurt, sugar substitute, and flaxseed meal.

2. Blend until smooth and creamy.

3. Add ice if desired for a colder smoothie.

4. Pour into a glass and serve chilled.

3. Tropical Paradise Smoothie:

Ingredients:

- 1/2 cup frozen pineapple chunks

- 1/2 cup frozen mango chunks

- 1/2 cup unsweetened coconut milk

- 1/4 cup unsweetened almond milk

- 1 tablespoon sugar substitute

- 1 tablespoon shredded coconut

Nutritional Value:

- Calories: 150

- Carbohydrates: 20g

- Protein: 2g

- Fat: 8g

- Fiber: 4g

Preparation:

1. In a blender, combine the frozen pineapple chunks, frozen mango chunks, coconut milk, almond milk, sugar substitute, and shredded coconut.

2. Blend until smooth and creamy.

3. Add ice if desired for a colder smoothie.

4. Serve chilled.

4. Peanut Butter Banana Smoothie:

Ingredients:

- 1 ripe banana

- 2 tablespoons natural peanut butter

- 1 cup unsweetened almond milk

- 1 tablespoon sugar substitute

- 1/2 teaspoon vanilla extract

Nutritional Value:

- Calories: 200

- Carbohydrates: 25g

- Protein: 7g

- Fat: 10g

- Fiber: 4g

Preparation:

1. In a blender, combine the ripe banana, peanut butter, almond milk, sugar substitute, and vanilla extract.

2. Blend until smooth and creamy.

3. Add ice if desired for a colder smoothie.

4. Serve chilled.

5. Chocolate Protein Shake:

Ingredients:

- 1 scoop chocolate protein powder

- 1 cup unsweetened almond milk

- 1 tablespoon unsweetened cocoa powder

- 1 tablespoon sugar substitute

- 1/2 teaspoon vanilla extract

Nutritional Value:

- Calories: 150

- Carbohydrates: 10g

- Protein: 20g

- Fat: 5g

- Fiber: 4g

Preparation:

1. In a blender, combine the chocolate protein powder, almond milk, cocoa powder, sugar substitute, and vanilla extract.

2. Blend until smooth and creamy.

3. Add ice if desired for a colder shake.

4. Serve chilled.

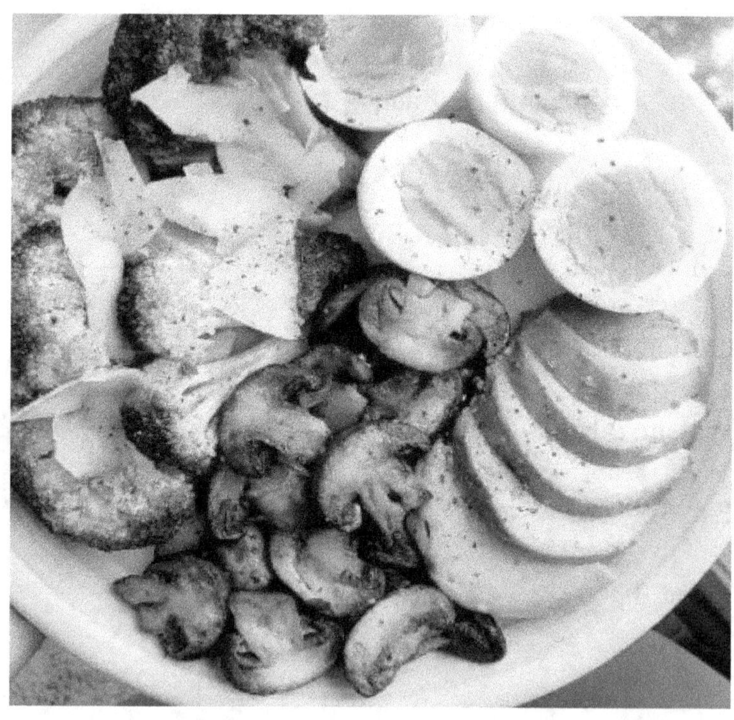

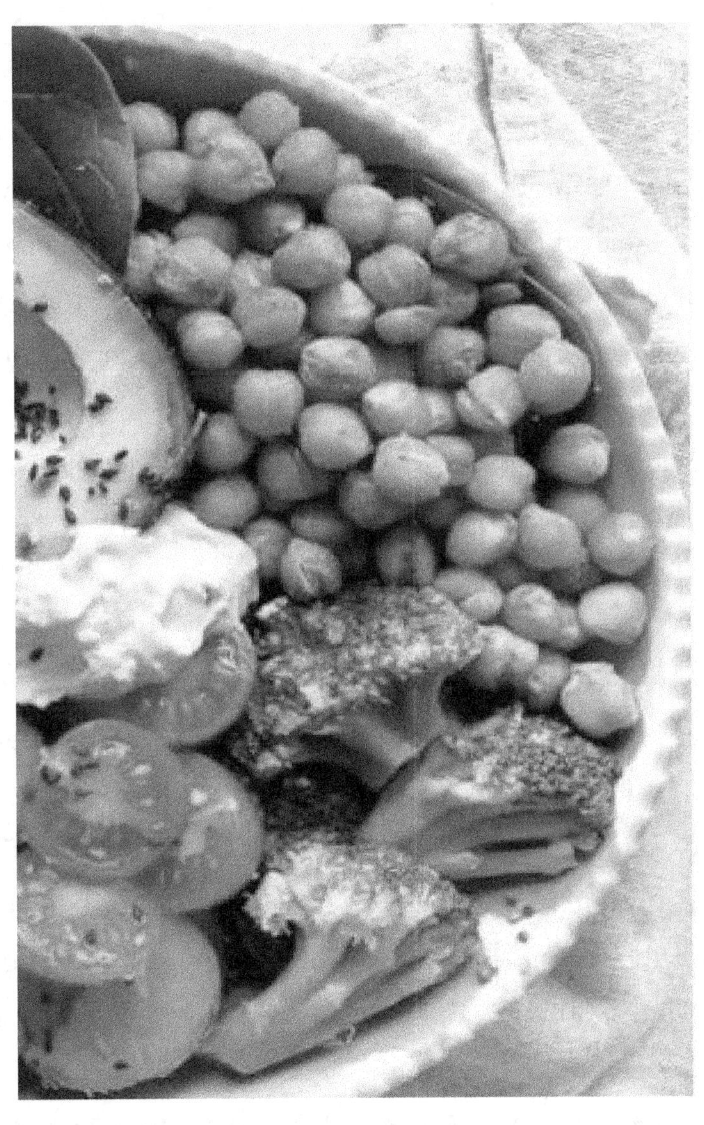

CHAPTER 6

Success Stories

Here I will like to share inspiring success stories of individuals who have successfully managed or even reversed their diabetes after the age of 50. These stories highlight the power of lifestyle changes and dietary choices in achieving optimal health and well-being. Get ready to be inspired and motivated by these real-life examples of individuals who took control of their diabetes and transformed their lives for the better.

John's Journey to Reversing Diabetes

John, a vibrant 55-year-old, was diagnosed with diabetes a few years ago. Determined to take charge of his health, he made significant lifestyle changes. He started incorporating regular exercise into his routine, such as brisk walking and strength training. John also focused on improving his diet by cutting out processed foods and sugary drinks, and instead opting for whole, nutrient-rich foods. With dedication and perseverance, John not only managed to control his blood sugar levels but also reversed his diabetes altogether. Today, he continues to maintain a healthy lifestyle and enjoys a life free from the constraints of diabetes.

Sarah's Success through Dietary Choices

Sarah, a 60-year-old grandmother, struggled with diabetes for many years. She decided to explore the power of dietary choices in managing her condition. Sarah adopted a low-carbohydrate diet, focusing on lean proteins, healthy fats, and plenty of vegetables. She limited her intake of refined sugars and processed grains, opting for whole grains instead. Through this dietary shift, Sarah experienced remarkable improvements in her blood sugar control. Her energy levels soared, and she even shed excess weight. Sarah's success story serves as a testament to the transformative effects of making mindful dietary choices.

Mark's Transformation through Lifestyle Changes

Mark, a 58-year-old retiree, was determined to improve his health after being diagnosed with diabetes. He decided to make comprehensive lifestyle changes that encompassed both diet and exercise. Mark started incorporating regular physical activity into his routine, including swimming and cycling. He also revamped his diet by focusing on portion control and incorporating more fruits, vegetables, and whole grains. Over time, Mark's dedication paid off as he witnessed significant improvements in his blood sugar levels and overall health. His success story showcases the power of holistic lifestyle changes in managing diabetes effectively.

These stories highlight the transformative power of lifestyle changes and dietary choices. Through dedication, perseverance, and making mindful decisions about exercise and nutrition, these individuals were able to take control of their diabetes and improve their overall health and well-being. Let these success stories serve as motivation and inspiration for your own journey towards optimal diabetes management. In the next chapter, we will delve into the importance of regular monitoring and self-care for maintaining long-term success.

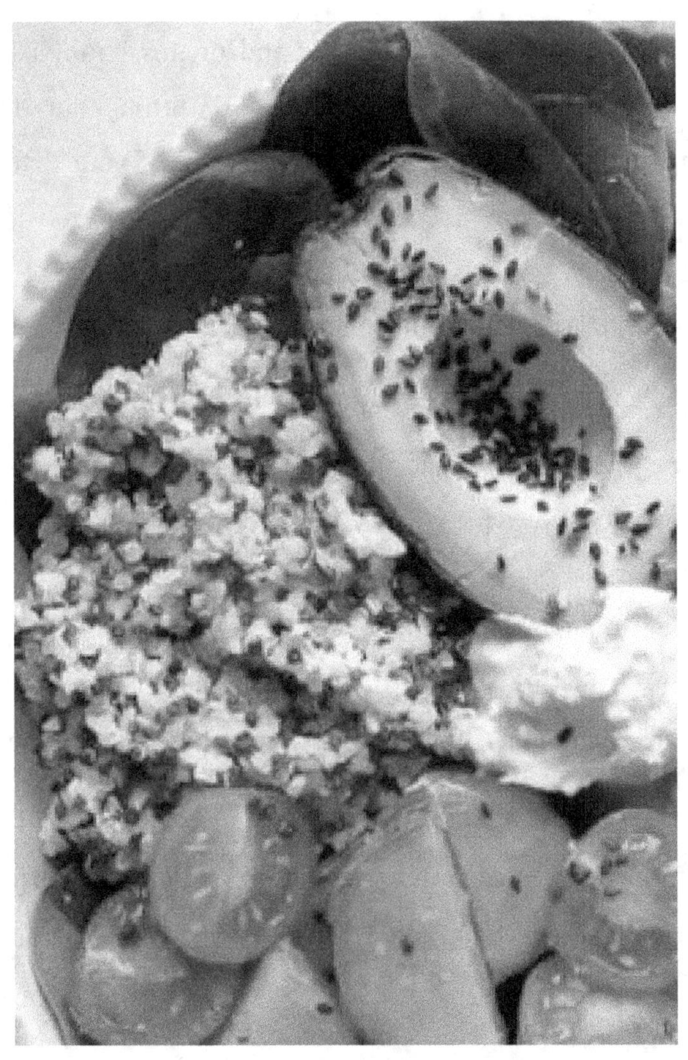

Conclusion

Congratulations on reaching the end of this book! I hope the stories and information shared throughout these chapters have inspired you to take control of your diabetes and make positive changes in your life. As you embark on this journey towards a healthier you, I want to leave you with a final message of hope and encouragement.

Managing and reversing diabetes after the age of 50 is not an easy task, but it is achievable. By incorporating regular exercise, improving your diet, and making mindful decisions about your overall well-being, you have the power to take control of your health and improve your quality of life. Remember, every small step you take towards a healthier lifestyle is a step in the right direction.

Reflecting on the journey of writing this book, I am grateful for the opportunity to share these valuable insights with you. I hope that my words have resonated with you and that you feel empowered to make positive changes in your life.

Adopting and adapting to this diabetic diet can have numerous benefits for individuals with diabetes. It can help improve blood sugar control, reduce the risk of complications associated with diabetes, and promote overall health and well-being. However, a balanced meal plan can aid weight management and support cardiovascular health.

To stay connected for my ongoing guidance, If you have any questions, I encourage you to send me an email via sheronjohnson@gmail.com. I will continue to provide valuable resources, tips, and support to help you on your journey towards a healthier you. Remember, you are not alone in this. I am here to support and cheer you on every step of the way.

Thank you for joining on this journey towards better health. I believe in you and wish you all the best as you continue on your path toward managing and preventing diabetes. Stay motivated, stay committed, and remember that you have the power to create a healthier and happier future for yourself.

HAPPY COOKING

Meal Planner Journal

Weekly
Diabetic diet Meal planner

Dates ______________

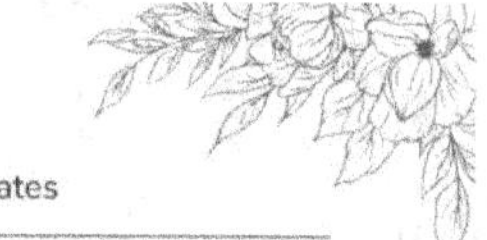

	BREAKFAST	LUNCH	DINNER	SNACKS
MON				
TUE				
WED				
THU				
FRI				
SAT				
SUN				

Shopping list

Weekly
Diabetic diet Meal planner

Dates ______________________

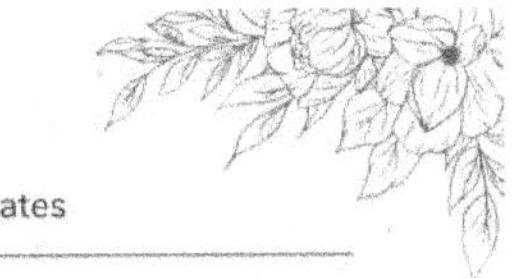

	BREAKFAST	LUNCH	DINNER	SNACKS
MON				
TUE				
WED				
THU				
FRI				
SAT				
SUN				

Shopping list

Weekly
Diabetic diet Meal planner

Dates ______________

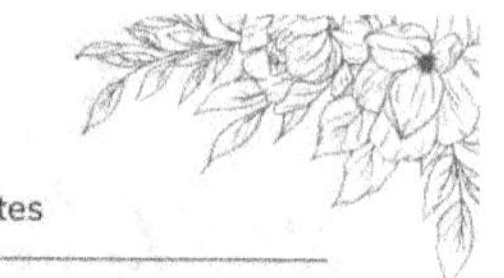

	BREAKFAST	LUNCH	DINNER	SNACKS
MON				
TUE				
WED				
THU				
FRI				
SAT				
SUN				

Shopping list

Weekly
Diabetic diet Meal planner

Dates ______________________

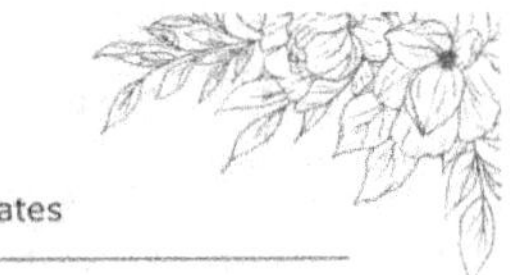

	BREAKFAST	LUNCH	DINNER	SNACKS
MON				
TUE				
WED				
THU				
FRI				
SAT				
SUN				

Shopping list

Weekly
Diabetic diet Meal planner

Dates ______________

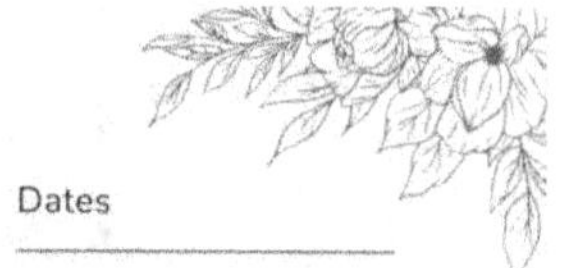

	BREAKFAST	LUNCH	DINNER	SNACKS
MON				
TUE				
WED				
THU				
FRI				
SAT				
SUN				

Shopping list

Weekly
Diabetic diet Meal planner

Dates
____

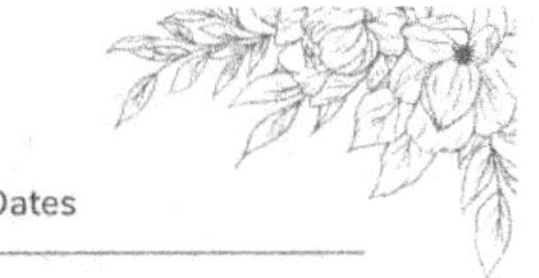

	BREAKFAST	LUNCH	DINNER	SNACKS
MON				
TUE				
WED				
THU				
FRI				
SAT				
SUN				

Shopping list

Weekly
Diabetic diet Meal planner

Dates ________________

	BREAKFAST	LUNCH	DINNER	SNACKS
MON				
TUE				
WED				
THU				
FRI				
SAT				
SUN				

Shopping list

Weekly
Diabetic diet Meal planner

Dates ___________________

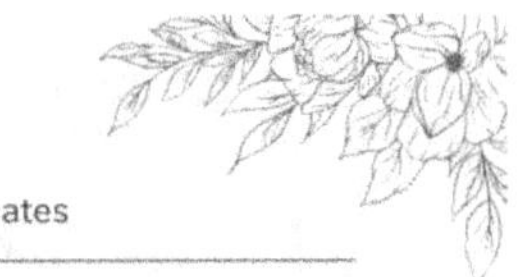

	BREAKFAST	LUNCH	DINNER	SNACKS
MON				
TUE				
WED				
THU				
FRI				
SAT				
SUN				

Shopping list

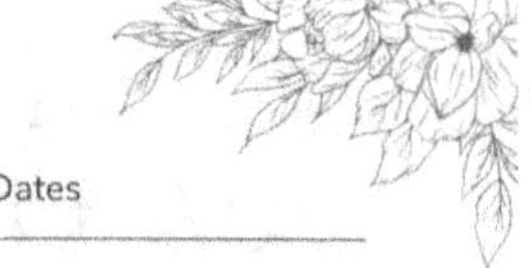

Weekly
Diabetic diet Meal planner

Dates ________________

	BREAKFAST	LUNCH	DINNER	SNACKS
MON				
TUE				
WED				
THU				
FRI				
SAT				
SUN				

Shopping list